SHEDDING
FOR THE WEDDING

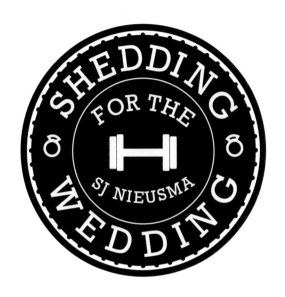

SHEDDING

FOR THE

SJ NIEUSMA

WEDDING

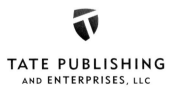

TATE PUBLISHING
AND ENTERPRISES, LLC

This book is designed to provide accurate and authoritative information with regard to the subject matter covered. This information is given with the understanding that neither the author nor Tate Publishing, LLC is engaged in rendering legal, professional advice. Since the details of your situation are fact dependent, you should additionally seek the services of a competent professional.

The opinions expressed by the author are not necessarily those of Tate Publishing, LLC.

Published by Tate Publishing & Enterprises, LLC
127 E. Trade Center Terrace | Mustang, Oklahoma 73064 USA
1.888.361.9473 | www.tatepublishing.com

Tate Publishing is committed to excellence in the publishing industry. The company reflects the philosophy established by the founders, based on Psalm 68:11,
"The Lord gave the word and great was the company of those who published it."

Book design copyright © 2012 by Tate Publishing, LLC. All rights reserved.
Cover design by Joel Uber
Interior design by Sarah Kirchen
Editing by Jevon Bolden, (Eric Nieusma) www.jevonbolden.com
Photography by Steve Kovich www.kovich.com
Illustration by Anna Horton Gainesville, FL

Published in the United States of America

ISBN: 978-1-61862-844-2
1. Health & Fitness / Women's Health
2. Health & Fitness / Weight Loss
12.04.17

This book is dedicated to the Lord, for giving me the idea of this book, for the passion for writing, and for all the books to come! Also, to all the soon-to-be brides who want to be their healthiest and fittest on their wedding day, this is for you!

"I can do all things through Christ who strengthens me," (Philippians 4:13, NKJV).

ACKNOWLEDGMENTS

I would like to thank my husband, Eric, for believing in me and also this book; for all of the support, encouragement, and time that he put into this book and into feeding my dreams!

TABLE OF CONTENTS

INTRODUCTION

Let me begin by saying, congratulations on your engagement. This is such an exciting and memorable time in your life. Having been a bride-to-be myself, I know how exciting yet hectic it can be when you finally sit down and begin the wedding checklist. On top of finding the perfect venue, the perfect caterer, the perfect cake, and the perfect photographer, you also want to find the perfect dress to seal the deal on your wedding day. But for some reason, you keep putting dress hunting off because you still know in the back of your mind that you want to shake some of the extra pounds you've been unhappily carrying around. You're wondering how to get into shape with a full-time job, meeting life's everyday demands, and managing to get at least eight hours of sleep every night, so you won't have those hateful bags under your eyes when the big day arrives. You wish there was a quick and easy way out.

That's where I come in! Being a former bride-to-be (as of August 14, 2010) and personal trainer, I have set up a fast, fun, and effective weight-loss program that will not only have you sweating for your wedding but also shedding fat for your wedding. This program will take no time at all and will produce the results you want and need for a healthier you. In less than thirty minutes a day, you will be able to fit this workout and diet into your busy schedule.

Are you ready for a healthier and sculpted you? Let's do this!

PS: There will be a wedding checklist to help guide you in your wedding planning with your weight loss listed as something that has to get done before the wedding day! I know you can do it!

INTERVAL TRAINING: BURNING FAT IN NO TIME

One thing a bride doesn't have a lot of is time. That is why this book is so helpful! With this program, you won't be spending countless hours in the gym. These workouts are short on time and tough on fat! Remembering how much time I didn't have when I was planning my wedding, I have put together an interval training program that's proven to blast more calories in *twenty minutes* than you would on the treadmill for sixty minutes. Here's how and why.

Interval training is not as complicated as it sounds. It's simply just alternating bursts of intense activity followed by much lighter activity or "recovery periods." This type of training can be used with any type of exercise.

Interval training is so effective for shedding fat because after you have completed your less-than-thirty-minute-interval workout, your body continues to burn calories and fat for two to four hours post-workout! In some cases, your body can keep burning calories for up to twenty-four hours, depending on the intensity of your intervals. In short, the harder your workouts are, the more calories you will burn. Research from the American College of Sport Medicine has shown that more calories are burned in short, high-intensity workouts than longer periods of cardio. "Traditional" cardio doesn't challenge the body's metabolism. In turn, you stop burning calories when you stop working out. You are going to do this three times per week in less than thirty minutes!

Remember This!

- Interval training burns more calories/fat in half the time of a traditional cardio work out where your heart rate stays the same.

- Interval training can raise your metabolism for up to twenty-four hours.

- Interval training can be up to ten times more effective than just cardio alone.

INTERVAL PROGRAMS

Interval training is the best way to burn fat and increase your overall level of fitness. Since I'm not there to determine your level of fitness, I want you to start at the beginner's level one and continue on from there. The first interval workout will be done two to three times a week in less than thirty minutes. At first your workout might only be fifteen minutes. If you want to do more, feel free! Remember to always warm up for about five minutes to get your blood flowing and help prevent injuries such as a muscle strain, sprains, or pull. (I will discuss warm-up options in more detail in chapter three.)

These workouts are all about giving a burst of your energy for a short period of time followed by a slightly longer time of slowing down, resting, or entering a recovery period. This puts your heart into a fat-burning zone. Just as you recover and catch your breath, you come out with another burst of energy followed by a recovery period. This is supposed to be difficult and strenuous to enforce fat burning. Once you have built up stamina and lungpower, you need to move on to harder intervals. Adding time onto the short period of energy bursts or cutting your rest time down will increase the difficulty. You never want to get used to a workout and stay there. It will create a plateau, and your weight loss will be at a standstill. Keep the intensity hard, and the weight will continue to fall off. You can use these interval workouts on the treadmill, bike, outdoor running, jump rope, elliptical, stepper, swimming, or any type of cardio that you enjoy doing. To make things easier on yourself, invest in an interval timer. It's a neat and inexpensive device that lets you program the interval periods in which you will be going strong in your workout and then recovering. It sounds a beep and lets you know when you have to start and stop. It's great if you're outside and don't have a watch.

Remember This!

- Interval training is short bursts of energy followed by recovery periods that are performed throughout the whole workout.

- If your body adapts to this workout, make it harder and avoid a plateau.

- By going hard and fast followed by rest or slower movement, your heart rate goes into what is called a fat-burning zone.

Now here is the basic structure of an interval workout:

- Workout 1

  - 5-minute warm-up
  - 20 seconds work, 40 seconds rest. Repeat this 5 times for a total of 5 minutes.
  - 5-minute cool down
  - 15 total minutes

- Workout 2

  - 5-minute warm-up
  - 20 seconds work, 40 seconds rest. Repeat this 7 times for a total of 7 minutes
  - 5-minute cool down
  - 17 total minutes

- Workout 3

  - 5-minute warm-up
  - 20 seconds work, 40 seconds rest. Repeat this 9 times for a total of 9 minutes
  - 5-minute cool down
  - 19 total minutes

- Workout 4
  - 5-minute warm-up
  - 20 seconds work, 40 seconds rest. Repeat this 11 times for a total of 11 minutes
  - 5-minute cool down
  - 21 total minutes
- Workout 5
  - 5-minute warm-up
  - 20 seconds work, 40 seconds rest. Repeat this 13 times for a total of 13 minutes
  - 5-minute cool down
  - 23 total minutes
- Workout 6
  - 5-minute warm-up
  - 20 seconds work, 40 seconds rest. Repeat this 15 times for a total of 15 minutes
  - 5-minute cool down
  - 25 total minutes

- Workout 7
  - 5-minute warm up
  - 20 seconds work, 40 seconds rest. Repeat this 17 times for a total of 17 minutes
  - 5-minute cool down
  - 27 total minutes
- Workout 8
  - 5-minute warm up
  - 20 seconds work, 40 seconds rest. Repeat this 19 times for a total of 19 minutes
  - 5-minute cool down
  - 29 total minutes

COMPOUND EXERCISES: SCULPTING YOUR BODY IN NO TIME

As the fat melts off your body from interval training, compound and superset training is its partner in crime by sculpting your physique and adding sleek shape to your body in no time. I chose these two powerful training methods because of the effect they have on fat burning, caloric expansion, and sculpting. There are multiple ways these exercises can be performed to prevent boredom and plateaus. Also, weight, sets, reps, and intensity can always be adjusted.

Compound exercises: weight training exercise that involves more than one joint and muscle group. An example of a compound exercise is a squat, which involves the joints of the knee, hip, and ankle and the muscles of the upper and lower legs and butt.

With compound exercises you are working multiple muscles versus just one muscle per exercise. This form of training helps burn more calories, allowing you to get a full-body workout fast. Compound training also benefits your coordination, reaction time, and balance. Compound exercises keep your heart rate up and provide cardiovascular benefit allowing you to exercise longer without muscle fatigue.

Remember This!

- Compound training is fast and effective in fat burning, caloric expansion, and sculpting.

- Compound training saves more time by letting you perform back-to-back exercises. A twenty-minute, two-to-three-times-a-week workout will do it!

- Compound training speeds up metabolism and is great for your heart!

YOUR SUPERSET AND COMPOUND WORKOUT PROGRAM

Compound exercises works more than one muscle group at a time, giving you the most benefit per exercise. I'm giving you twelve different compound (workouts) exercises. You are only going to train like this two to three days a week. If at first you can only do this one day a week, don't worry. You will be able to work up to three days a week! I have created each program to sculpt three to four muscle groups in one session. Each workout is already mapped out for you, so all you have to do is follow my lead!

Remember to warm up for five to ten minutes before working out. A good warm-up is complete when you have broken a sweat! Jogging in place, taking a slow run, jumping jacks, riding a bike, and the like are all acceptable warm-ups.

Once you are warmed up, get ready to move fast through this workout, because I am giving you short periods of rest in between each exercise to ensure optimum fat burning and caloric expansion. All you will need is a set of dumbbells for these workouts. This is a great benefit for you to spend minimal money on equipment and avoid costly gym memberships.

Since I'm not there to help you select a weight that is good for you to work out with, purchase a set of dumbbells that you can curl or press over your head between fifteen to twenty times. For most women this will be between five- to twelve-pound weights. If you can get to fifteen reps with no problem, then up the weight! We will be typically doing fifteen to twenty-plus reps in this program, so you want to make sure that by the time you hit your tenth rep, your muscle is burning and you have to push yourself to get to fifteen or twenty reps.

Remember, we don't want this to feel easy. Your last rep should be difficult but not impossible. You can perform each program three to five days a week, depending upon your fitness goals, determination, and ability.

YOUR COMPOUND PROGRAM

MONDAY'S COMPOUND WORKOUT

Perform the four compound exercises below back-to-back (without resting), doing fifteen to twenty-five reps per exercise. After completing fifteen to twenty-five reps for all of Monday's exercises, rest for one to two minutes and repeat three times. Breathing will be labeled "inhale" and "exhale." During the inhale you want to tighten your stomach and breathe in through your nose. During the exhale you want to blow out slowly through your mouth.

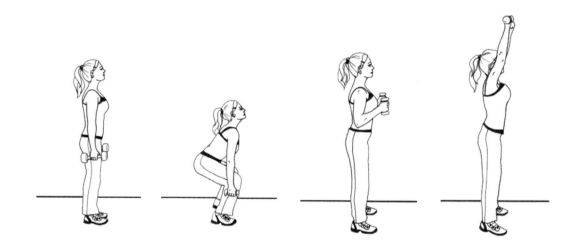

This exercise will tone the lower body, arms, and shoulders.

SQUAT, CURL, PRESS

Step 1: Stand straight up with weights to your side. Inhale.

Step 2: Keeping your back straight, slowly sit back as if a chair were behind you, allowing your knees to bend.

Step 3: Return to standing position and curl the weights at the same time while exhaling.

Step 4: Press the weights over your head.

Do's: Keep back straight and weight under your heels while squatting

Don'ts: Don't allow knees to go over toes when squatting

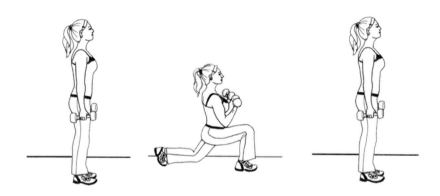

This exercise will tone the legs, butt, and arms.

LUNGE AND CURL

Step 1: Stand straight up with weights to your side. Inhale.

Step 2: Take one big step forward and drop straight down keeping your back straight. Drop down until your back knee is almost touching the floor.

Step 3: Press off your forward heel and return to starting position while curling weight. Exhale.

Do's: Keep back straight, and lunge with each leg the same number of times.

Don'ts: Don't let your knee go over your toe on forward leg. Don't use weight if the lunge is too difficult.

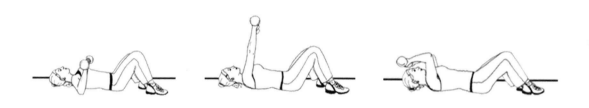

This exercise strengthens the chest and tones the back upper arm.

CHEST PRESS AND TRICEP EXTENSION

Step 1: Lie on a flat surface with your knees bent, arms away from your body, elbows bent. Inhale.

Step 2: Press the weight directly over your chest. Exhale.

Step 3: Inhale. Allow your elbow to bend and take weights back to the sides of your ears. Extend elbow back so weight are over your chest. Exhale.

Do's: Keep a firm grip on the weight.

Don'ts: Don't press the weight or take it back over your face at any time.

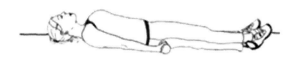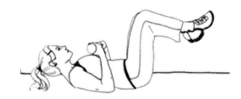

This exercise will tighten the midsection and tone arms.

CRUNCH AND CURL

Step 1: Lie on flat surface with arms to side palms up and legs straight. Inhale small breath and tighten stomach muscles.

Step 2: Bring knees toward chest, curl arms up, keeping elbows on flat surface, and squeeze abs and exhale slowly.

Do's: Keep your stomach tight while performing this exercise.

Don'ts: Touch your chin to chest

WEDNESDAY'S COMPOUND WORKOUT

Perform the four compound exercises below back-to-back (without resting), doing fifteen to twenty-five reps per exercise. After completing fifteen to twenty-five reps for all of Wednesday's exercises, rest for one to two minutes and repeat three times. Breathing will be labeled, "inhale" and "exhale." During the inhale you want to tighten your stomach and breathe in through your nose. During the exhale you want to blow out slowly through your mouth.

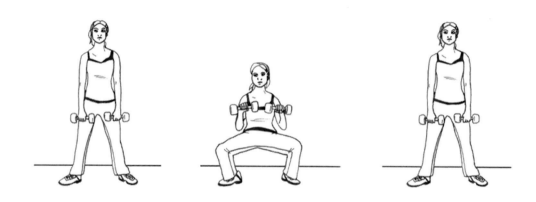

This exercise will tighten your butt and tone your arms.

SUMO SQUAT AND REVERSE CURL

Step 1: Stand straight up, feet spread wide apart, holding weights to your side with your palms facing backward. Inhale.

Step 2: Keeping your back straight, slowly sit back as if a chair were behind you, allowing your knees to bend.

Step 3: Return to starting position. Curl the weights at the same time, keeping the reverse grip. Exhale.

Do's: Keep back straight and weight under your heels while squatting.

Don'ts: Don't allow knees to go over toes when squatting.

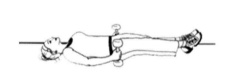
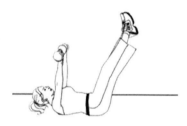

This exercise will tighten your midsection and tone shoulders.

LEG AND SHOULDER RAISE

Step 1: Lie on a flat surface arms at your side legs extended. Inhale, tighten stomach.

Step 2: Raise arms and legs at the same time, keeping them both straight. Raise arms until weights are over chest, and raise legs until the bottom of your feet are facing the ceiling. Exhale during the movement.

Do's: Keep abs tight while lifting your legs.

Don'ts: Don't hold your breath.

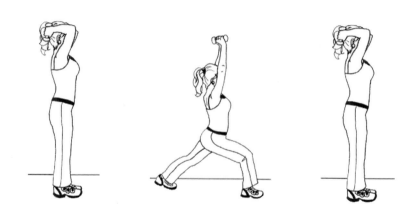

This exercise will tone the legs, butt, and arms.

LUNGE AND TRICEP EXTENSION

Step 1: Stand straight up with the weight behind your head, elbows bent. Inhale.

Step 2: Take one big step forward and drop straight down, keeping your back straight. Drop down until your back knee is almost touching the floor.

Step 3: Press off your forward heel and return to starting position while extending your arms so the weight is over your head. Exhale.

Do's: Keep back straight; lunge with each leg the same number of times.

Don'ts: Don't let your knee go over your toe on forward leg. Don't use weight if the lunge is too difficult.

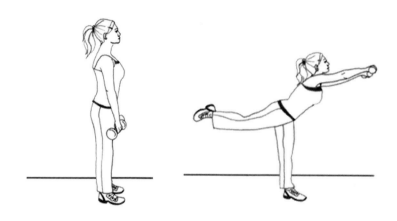

This exercise will tone the butt, back, and arms.

LEG EXTENSION AND RAISE

Step 1: Stand straight up with weights to your side. Inhale.

Step 2: Keeping your legs straight, take one leg back until the top of your foot is facing the floor and raise your arms until the weights are eye level. Exhale.

Do's: Keep a flat back or slightly arch it backward.

Don'ts: Don't use weights if you have trouble balancing.

FRIDAY'S COMPOUND WORKOUT

Perform the four compound exercises below back-to-back (without resting), doing fifteen to twenty-five reps per exercise. After completing fifteen to twenty-five reps for all of Friday's exercises, rest for one to two minutes and repeat three times. Breathing will be labeled "inhale" and "exhale." During the inhale you want to tighten your stomach and breathe in through your nose. During the exhale you want to blow out slowly through your mouth.

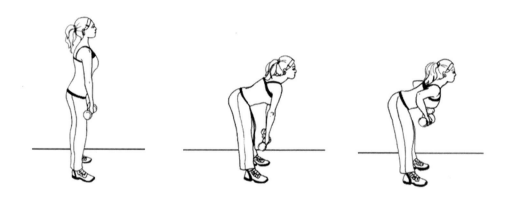

This exercise will tone your legs, butt, and upper and lower back.

STIFF LEG LIFT AND ROW

Step 1: Stand straight up with a small bend in your knees; hold weights to your side. Inhale.

Step 2: Bend over like you are going to touch your toes while keeping your back straight. Go down until your belly button is facing the floor; return to standing upright while exhaling.

Step 3: Inhale. While keeping your arms straight, thumbs facing up, raise the weights in front of you to shoulder level; exhale, and return weights to your side.

Do's: Keep your back straight or slightly arched backward while bending over

Don'ts: Don't round your back when bending over

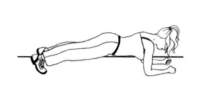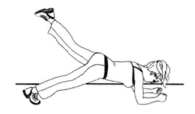

This exercise will tone your midsection and butt.

CORE PLANK AND LEG EXTENSION

Step 1: Get into a pushup position with your forearms flat on the ground

Step 2: Keeping your legs straight, lift one heel toward the ceiling until it can't go any further then return the foot to the ground. Alternate legs each rep.

Do's: If the exercise is too hard on the floor, try it with your arms on an elevated surface, like a bed. Breathe regularly throughout this exercise; counting your reps out loud is a good way to regulate your breathing. Keep your back flat.

Don'ts: Don't let your back sag toward the ground.

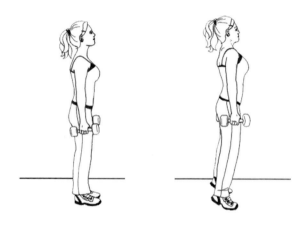

This exercise will strengthen your lower leg and shoulders.

HEEL RAISE AND SHRUG

Step 1: Stand straight up with weights to your side. Inhale.

Step 2: Lift your heels off the ground by going up on your toes, and raise your shoulders at the same time. Exhale.

Do's: Perform this exercise with a wall behind you in case you lose your balance. To make the exercise more difficult, stand on one foot while performing the heel raises.

Don'ts: Don't hold your breath.

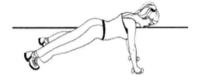 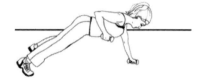

This exercise will tone your midsection and back.

CORE PLANK AND BACK ROW

Step 1: Get in a pushup position with your feet spread wide and your hands on the dumbbells

Step 2: Lift one weight of the floor by taking your elbow backwards and up until it is even

Do's: Try this exercise without weights first. If it's too hard on the floor, try it with your hands on an elevated surface, like a bed. Breathe regularly throughout this exercise; counting your reps out loud is a good way to regulate your breathing. Keep your back flat

Don'ts: Don't let your back sag toward the ground.

NUTRITION 80

Ladies, this is the most important chapter in this book. Here I will be giving you a grocery list, food index, and optional food log to help get you on track to form good habits that will lead to your success. The chapter is called Nutrition 80 because when working toward your weight-loss goals, diet stands at 80 percent of the 100 percent that will determine the outcome of your tight physique. Have you ever heard the expression "abs are made in the kitchen"? Well they are! The last 20 percent is made up of exercise and genetics both standing at 10 percent each. Yes, working out is only 10 percent of your physique's final outcome, but that doesn't mean you don't have to work out! You are sculpting your body and creating a sleek shape when you lift weights. So let's get started on changing your life forever!

With all the fad diets out nowadays, I can't figure out why people aren't getting the point that they don't work! Often people who try these fad diets lose weight quickly. But after the weight falls off, they just fall back into their old eating habits because new healthy eating habits weren't created or formed. In fact, forty-five million people go on a diet every year, and with ninety-seven million Americans overweight, something has got to change! Well, I have the answer, and it's very simple—eat healthy, frequently, and get your proportions right. Yes, it is that easy!

A clean diet consists of the right carbs, lean proteins, and healthy fats. Eating healthy will not only help you achieve success with your fat loss, but it will also fuel you with food energy to get you through each day. Eating clean is best described as foods that are free of manmade sugars, hydrogenated fats, trans fats, and other harmful preservatives.

Here are a few examples of bad eating habits and things to avoid that will lead to weight gain and a slow metabolism.

- Not eating enough and not eating at the right times

- Eating the wrong foods and portion sizes

- Fad diets opposed to healthy eating

- Waiting until you're hungry or starving to eat

First things first: breakfast, also known as "breaking the fast," is the *most* important meal of the day! Why is eating breakfast so important? While sleeping, your metabolism slows down. After a certain amount of time (getting up and not eating until lunchtime, for example), your body goes into what's called "starvation mode." This is where your body reacts to the absence of food and begins to store fat in fear that food will not be coming in anytime soon. This is why it's imperative to get up and eat something that will get your metabolism revved up and give you energy. That alone will kick you into weight-loss mode.

The next important factor in losing weight and keeping it off is eating frequently. Eating smaller portions every three hours or so will keep your energy level up, cravings at bay, and your metabolism kicked into high gear. Basically you want to have breakfast, lunch, and dinner with healthy snacks in between. Eating throughout the day keeps your body at work by having to constantly break down food instead of getting it in one or two big meals each day. Eating frequently will also help balance blood sugar levels making you feel healthier, fuller, and reduce those cravings to eat something you shouldn't. When we don't eat at the times we should, our bodies begin to crave any and everything. It's a vicious cycle.

Now that you're eating more frequently, let's talk about what foods you should be eating and why. First off, drink plenty of water. Drink eight to ten glasses a day, and when working out, you will need more. Water helps to flush your system out and also aids in weight loss. Dr. Oz suggests that drinking a large glass of cold water before you eat a meal will help cut down on unnecessary calories. At every meal you should try and have a lean protein, complex carbohydrates, and healthy fats. Eating the combination of these three will enable the body to utilize and absorb the nutrients from food to be used for maximum efficiency. Proteins, carbs, and fats make the perfect balance of nutrition to feed your muscles, give you energy, and assist in healthy-looking skin and hair.

You also want to make sure you are getting the natural sugars into your diet that consists of any type of fruit you like. White or artificial sugars are extremely harmful to your physique and health. They are found in any candy, soda, cookie, or ice cream.

Lean protein is used in the body to build, maintain, and replace tissue, including muscles, hair, skin, nails, organs, and glands. Complex carbs are the primary source for energy in the body. Healthy fats help vitamins A, D, E, and K absorb into our bodies and are great for your heart and menstrual cycle!

Stay away from junk food as much as possible. Fried food and sweets will slow down your weight loss. Treat yourself once a week (if you have to), and remember to eat any junk food in moderation. It won't kill you if your diet is healthy 99 percent of the time.

Remember This!

- Never skip breakfast! Break the fast and eat frequently.

- Stick to lean proteins, complex carbohydrates, and healthy fats at each meal.

- Stay away from refined sweets, sodas, and fried foods.

- Drink plenty of water.

- Eat before you have a hunger attack.

GROCERY LIST

This grocery list is broken up into lean proteins, complex carbohydrates, healthy fats, and natural sugars. Try to make sure you always have a couple of foods from each group listed in your kitchen. This will ensure your success by always having the right combination of food on hand. Drink plenty of water!

LEAN PROTEINS:

- Chicken breast
- Egg whites
- Turkey breast
- All white tuna in water
- Fish (tilapia, salmon, mahi mahi, cod, or tuna)
- Fat-free cheese
- Lean beef (hamburger meat and lean steak once a week for iron intake)
- Low-fat cottage cheese
- Tofu- Vegan
- Quinoa- Vegan

- Gimmie Lean (sausage)- Vegan
- Veggie Burgers- Vegan
- Smart Dogs- Vegan
- Tofurkey- Vegan
- Quinoa- Vegan

COMPLEX CARBOHYDRATES:

- Brown rice
- Sweet potatoes
- Red potatoes
- Whole-wheat bread
- Whole-wheat bagels or whole-wheat English muffins
- Lentils
- Beans (black, pinto, Kidney)
- Wheat pasta
- Quinoa

HEALTHY FATS:

- Olive oil
- (Grapeseed oil)
- Nuts (almonds, walnuts)
- Flax seed
- Avocado
- Guacamole

NATURAL SUGARS:

- Any fruit (strawberries, blueberries, apples, pears, plums, grapes, bananas)
- Honey (raw is the best)
- Agave
- Unsweetened applesauce

VEGETABLES:

- Any and every kind is good to have in your home

STRESS CORTISOL EXPOSED

Let's face it, stress is inevitable, but the amount of stress we take in is not! The reason I'm choosing to inform you about the side effects of stress is because weight gain is one of them. While planning your wedding, stress will arise, so hopefully you can take this information and give stress the back seat to your wedding planning!

The culprit in the weight gain or absence of weight loss in the occurrence of stress is a hormone produced in the adrenal glands called cortisol. The body naturally produces a low level of cortisol that is not harmful. When you are under stress, the body produces an unhealthy amount of cortisol by converting protein into glucose (sugar). It basically gives your body the energy to go into battle or fight off a stressful situation. Not only can cortisol dip into muscle growth by breaking it down, but it also leaves your blood sugar level dangerously high. Here is where the weight gain takes place. We don't end up using all the converted glucose, and the rest of it gets left in the body and inevitably turns into fat. Crazy, right?

Also, there are other negative side effects from stress. When cortisol is produced in your body at a higher rate due to stress, it raises your blood sugar from all the glucose! It also raises your blood pressure and suppresses your immune system. Scientist Hans Selye, who introduced the General Adaption Syndrome in 1936 concerning stress, states that "Stress also contributes to high blood pressure, heart disease, rheumatoid arthritis, and other stress related illness." I'm sure you don't want to be sick on your wedding day. So basically, stress is the enemy.

The great thing about exercising and eating healthy is together they help keep stress at bay. When exercising, your body produces endorphins that give you a happy feeling or natural high. It's terrific for fighting off stress and can actually fight off depression! When eating healthy, you aren't left with a feeling of guilt from eating junk, and stress is less likely to attack your mind.

When you find yourself experiencing stress, try to do an extra workout that I have given you. Not only will you burn more calories, but you will also release those good-feeling endorphins! You'll also benefit for a big feeling of accomplishment! The workouts take no time at all, so that means the feeling of stress will also be gone in no time!

Remember This!

- When under stress, the body produces cortisol, turning protein into sugar, which then turns into fat!

- Cortisol raises blood sugar, blood pressure, and suppresses your immune system.

- Exercising produces endorphins (natural high) that help fight stress!

SUPPLEMENTS FOR THE ACTIVE WOMAN

Vitamins and minerals are important for everyone, at any age, active or not. Because you are now considered an active woman, it's time for you to be informed on the proper vitamins, minerals, antioxidants, and daily supplements your body needs. Even though your new, healthy eating will be giving you vitamins from what's naturally found in food, your body requires more when you increase your activity level. Here is a list of vitamins and an explanation on why they are so needed!

- Vitamin A: Is good for your eyes, healing wounds, and supporting your immune system.

- Vitamin B: Fights fatigue and the symptoms of PMS. Also folic acid, which is a B vitamin, is important for women when pregnant.

- Vitamin C: Helps support immune system, keeps skin healthy and young, and reduces the risk of cancer and tissue damage.

- Vitamin D: Is good for proper absorption of calcium, prevents osteoporosis, and is great for healthy joints. Professor of medicine at Boston University states, "Vitamin D reduces blood pressure: It decreases the production of a hormone called renin, which is believed to play a role in hypertension."

- Vitamin E: Reduces the risk of heart disease, is an antioxidant, and protects the red blood cells.

- Antioxidants: The vitamins, minerals, and enzymes that may protect your body from diseases such as cancer, heart disease, stroke, rheumatoid arthritis, and Alzheimer's disease. They protect the body by destroying free radicals (harmful cells or cancerous cells). Vitamins A, C, and E are also found in fruit. It's important to have antioxidants and vitamins after a workout to help repair tissue and cell damage.

- Omegas 3, 6, and 9: Essential fatty acids are necessary for good health. A polyunsaturated fat is a good fat that helps in heart health, brain function, lowers blood pressure, helps with the symptoms of PMS, and helps fight depression. Omegas 3, 6, and 9 are also great for hair and skin.

- Calcium: Is an essential mineral with a wide range of roles. As one of the most important minerals, calcium is important for bone health, proper immune function, muscle contraction, and much more. It's so important that the National Academy of Science has established a standard that women between the ages of twenty to fifty should take 1,000 mg of calcium a day, and women over fifty should take 1,200 mg a day.

- Iron: Is a very important vitamin for women due to the loss of it during our menstrual cycle. When our bodies lack iron, we may feel tired, sluggish, and can bruise easily. Iron can help prevent cancer, improve the body's energy level, protect your immune system, and also help decrease the symptoms of insomnia.

- Protein shake: Great for weight management by helping the body feel fuller longer. Protein helps in repairing damaged muscle tissue after a workout. Protein is known as a "macronutrient," which means the body needs relatively large amounts of it to maintain optimum health. Hair and nails are made up of mostly protein, and it's needed to make enzymes, hormones, and other bodily chemicals. Protein is important for cartilage, skin, bones, and blood.

- Try to get a soy or whey protein shake that is low in fat and carbs. Soy is from plant protein, and whey is from animal protein, so you have a choice. There is a wide variety of flavor choices ranging from Dutch chocolate, vanilla, banana cream, strawberry, and more! They also make great protein smoothies with a little fruit and ice added. Drink the protein shake within thirty minutes post-workout to help build lean muscle and fight fat.

You can get all of these supplements for a very low price at www.BuildingBrawn.com. These supplements are very important. They will aid in your weight loss while keeping your body strong, fit, and healthy.

RECIPES FOR HEALTHY AND DELICIOUS PROTEIN SMOOTHIES!

This chapter is filled with healthy protein-packed smoothies to help you fuel up before your workout and replenish you after your workouts. These smoothies are best consumed post-workout because they have protein to help rebuild broken-down muscle fibers. Fruit has carbohydrates and simple sugars to replenish your glycogen storages. Also, Matcha green tea is best for fighting off free radicals with its powerful antioxidants! These super-strong antioxidants are also great for reducing signs of aging and help fight off diseases such as cancer. Matcha tea can be enjoyed alone or by having it in the smoothie. The most important time to drink these smoothies is after your work out because you need to give your body the proper nutrition to burn the fat and build the muscle!

It's up to you whether you want to prepare the fruit fresh or frozen. Whatever texture suits you best! With all the milk ingredients, I recommend using nut milks; i.e., almond or coconut, but feel free to use dairy or soy.

STRAWBERRY GREEN TEA PROTEIN SMOOTHIE

INGREDIENTS:

1 tsp Tea Trim Matcha
1 cup strawberries (fresh or frozen)
1/2 cup fat-free Greek yogurt
1 scoop protein powder (vanilla)
How to Make: Put all ingredients into blender and mix.
Nutrition Facts:
Calories: 135
Total fat: 3 g.
Total carbs: 16 g.
Protein: 23 g.

PEANUT BUTTER-ALMOND-BANANA SMOOTHIE

INGREDIENTS:

1 banana

1 scoop vanilla or chocolate protein powder

1 cup (skim) almond milk

1 tbsp. natural peanut butter

3 ice cubes

How to Make: Mix all ingredients in a blender and mix.

Nutritional Facts:

Calories: 217

Total fat: 7 g.

Total carbs: 40 g.

Protein: 25 g.

TROPICAL FRUIT SMOOTHIE

INGREDIENTS:

1/2 mango
5 strawberries
1/2 banana
1 cup of water
1 scoop of vanilla protein powder
How to Make: Put all ingredients in blender and mix
Nutritional Facts:
Calories: 200
Total fat: 4 g.
Total carbs: 31 g.
Protein: 32 g.

PEACH PARADISE SMOOTHIE

INGREDIENTS:

1/2 peach
1 cup of almond milk
1/4 cup of soft tofu
Handful of ice
1 packet of stevia
1 scoop vanilla protein powder
How to Make: Peel peach. Put all ingredients in blender and mix.
Nutritional Facts:
Calories: 181
Total fat: 1 g.
Total carbs: 20 g.
Protein: 23 g.

BLUEBERRY-PINEAPPLE SMOOTHIE

INGREDIENTS:

1/2 cup of blueberries
1/2 cup pineapple, diced
8 oz. low-fat Greek yogurt
2 tsp. of sweetener
1 scoop vanilla protein powder
1/2 cup water
How to Make: Put all ingredients in blender and mix.
Nutritional Facts:
Calories: 246
Total fat: 2 g.
Total carbs: 31 g.
Protein: 26 g.

COFFEE CHOCOLATE–BANANA SMOOTHIE

INGREDIENTS:

1 banana
1 cup low-fat milk
8 oz. low-fat coffee yogurt
1/4 teaspoon of cinnamon
1 packet sweetener
Dash of nutmeg
How to Make: Peel banana. Mix all ingredients in a blender and mix.
Nutritional Facts:
Calories: 178
Total fat: 2 g.
Total carbs: 48 g.
Protein: 28 g.

MATCHA BERRY GOODNESS SMOOTHIE

INGREDIENTS:

1 cup berries (whatever kind you like)
1/2 banana
1/2 cup of milk
1/3 cup of low-fat yogurt
Handful of ice
1 scoop of vanilla or strawberry protein powder
1 tsp Tea Trim Matcha tea
How to Make: Put all ingredients in blender and mix.
Nutritional Facts:
Calories: 274
Total fat: 0 g.
Total carbs: 58 g.
Protein: 31 g.

STRAWBERRY-MANGO MATCHA MADNESS SMOOTHIE

INGREDIENTS:

1/2 mango
1 cup skim milk
1/4 tbsp. vanilla extract
1 scoop vanilla protein powder
1 tsp Tea Trim Matcha tea
Handful of ice
How to Make: Peel mango and chop. Put all ingredients in blender and mix.
Nutritional Facts:
Calories: 412
Total fat: 4.2 g.
Total carbs: 54 g.
Protein: 28 g.

SWEET CHERRY-CANTALOUPE SMOOTHIE

INGREDIENTS:

1/2 cup cantaloupe
1/2 cup of apples
3 cherries
1/4 cup raspberries
Handful of ice cubes
1 scoop vanilla protein powder
How to Make: Peel and chop cantaloupe. Put all ingredients in blender and mix.
Nutritional Facts:
Calories: 278
Total fats: 4 g.
Total carbs: 28 g.
Protein: 31 g.

FAT-FREE VANILLA STRAWBERRY-BANANA SMOOTHIE

INGREDIENTS:

1/2 banana
10 strawberries
Handful of ice
1/2 cup water
1 scoop vanilla protein powder
How to Make: Put all ingredients in blender and mix.
Nutritional Facts:
Calories: 209
Total Fat: 0 g.
Total Carbs: 25 g.
Protein: 27 g.

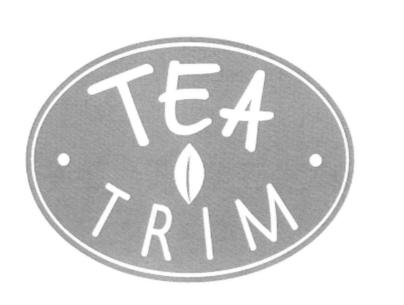

TEA TRIM

Tea Trim Matcha is the perfect aid in reaching your weight-loss goals. It raises metabolism, increases fat oxidation, curves appetite, increases endurance, and helps prevent fat from absorbing. Those using Tea Trim matcha regularly can burn four times the calories per workout. Tea Trim is best to take thirty minutes before exercise to help increase endurance and burn fat. Tea Trim Matcha consumption has to be consistent in order to be efficient.
   Tea Trim Matcha Benefits

- Burn fat—boost metabolism and oxidize fat quicker

- Fight cancer and disease with powerful antioxidants EGCg, vitamins, and minerals

- Slows aging—Naturally detox and cleanse with chlorophyll; antioxidants protect collagen breakdown, promote relaxation, and reduce stress

- Boost Energy mentally and physically. Boost your daily motivation level and workout routines

- Tea Trim Matcha is 100% USDA organic, sugar free, RAW, vegan friendly, gluten free, soy free, dairy free, Non GMO, and has no artificial colors, flavors, preservatives, chemicals, pesticides, or additives.

- Tea Trim Matcha has ten times the antioxidants as pomegranates and blueberries

- One glass of Tea Trim matcha is the equivalent of ten glasses of green tea in terms of nutritional value and antioxidant content.

- Excellent Choice for Diabetics; Matcha is a zero on the Glycemic index

- Tea Trim's Matcha will give you a trimmer midsection by cleaning the fat-storing toxins with high chlorophyll content.

- Use as a skin prep in your beauty regimen for a glowing look on your wedding day

- Purchase Tea Trim at www.teatrim.com

TIPS FOR SUCCESS

When changing your lifestyle to a more active and healthy one, lack of things like planning, timing, and pre-organizing can be the main reasons why failure occurs. Here are some fail-proof tips in securing your success.

NUTRITION TIPS

- Stick to the outside of the grocery store where the fruits, vegetables, meats, and dairy are as much as possible. Always have a food list planned, and stick to it.

- Always make sure your kitchen is stalked up with the right foods.

- Make meals and snacks on Sunday for the following week. Have the correct proportions of food and put them in small containers. This way all you have to do is grab your food and go!

- Try to buy the food you will be eating a lot of in bulk. This saves money and another trip to the grocery store. Try and freeze some of the veggies and lean protein to keep food from going bad.

- Try and switch up your fruits, veggies, and lean protein every week or every other week. This way you can look forward to having something new and won't get sick of the same old thing. Variety is the key.

- When cooking, try to use a fat free, non-stick spray to eliminate extra fat in your diet.

- When baking, use Truvia, Stevia, or agave for natural sugar substances.

- Fill out the food log for the first week to keep track of your nutrition (see Appendix C). This will enable you to see where you have missed a meal or eaten something you shouldn't have. This way you can get back on track fast.

EXERCISE TIPS

- Always remember to warm up before you workout and cool down after. Also don't forget to stretch.

- Drink plenty of water before, during, and after a workout.

- If the workouts begin to get too easy, adjust your intensity, increase speed, increase the free weight amount, and even add more time on to the workout. Don't let your body get used to any type of workout. Your progress will stop there. It will plateau.

- Wear sneakers that support your ankles and are comfortable.

- If you're really sore, allow those muscles to rest, and take a day or more off from working out.

- Have a mental idea of where and what time you will be working out. Make it a priority. Try exercising in the morning to boost energy levels during the day.

- Get a workout buddy. It's always better when you have someone working as hard as you are.

STRESS MANAGEMENT TIPS

- Find a yoga class and take it weekly. It will help your whole body and mind to relax.

- Work on breathing exercises. Sometimes that's all we need to calm our mind.

- Don't ingest a lot of caffeine. It enhances emotions, and if stress is already present, it will only make it worse.

- Go to a comedy club or rent a funny movie. Laughter is nature's medicine.

- Go for a walk outdoors. The fresh air and sounds of nature are relaxing.

- Get a massage, pedicure, or manicure with your friends.

- Meditate on the positive. Envision your weight loss. Think of finding your perfect wedding dress and even pretend you are on your honeymoon, and take a mental vacation.

- Do an extra workout and feel those endorphins. This has a long-term effect of self-satisfaction.

- Read a book.

APPENDIX A:
NUTRITIONALFOOD COUNTS

1   2   3

NUTRITION FOOD COUNTS – CARBOHYDRATES

Food	Carbs	Fat	Protein	Calories
Oatmeal ½ cup	27 grams - 4 fiber	3 grams- .5 Sat	5 grams	155 kcal
Sweet potato 2oz	15 grams - 2 fiber	0 grams	1 gram	64 kcal
Sweet potato 4oz	30 grams - 4 fiber	0 grams	2 grams	128 kcal
Sweet potato 6 oz	45 grams - 6 fiber	0 grams	3 grams	192 kcal
Sweet potato 8oz	60 grams- 8 fiber	0 grams	4 grams	256 kcal
½ cup brown rice cooked	22 grams- 2 fiber	1 gram	2.5 grams	108 kcal

Brown rice cooked 1 cup	44grams- 2 fiber	2 grams	5 grams	216 kcal
½ cup pinto beans cooked	22 grams- 6 fiber	1 gram	8 grams	129 kcal
Lentils ¼ cup dry	19 grams- 9 fiber	0 grams	8 grams	70 kcal
Wheat bread 1 slice	10 grams- 2 fiber	1 gram	4 grams	70 k cal
Wheat pasta	42grams- 2 fiber	1 gram	7 grams	210 kcal
Light red kidney beans	22 carbs- 14 fiber	0 grams	9 grams	70 kcal
Quinoa ½ cup cooked	20 grams- 2.5 fiber	2 grams	4 grams	111 kcal
Couscous ½ cup cooked	18 grams- 1 fiber	0 grams	3 grams	88 kcal

NUTRITION FOOD COUNTS - FATS

Food	Carbs	Fat	Protein	Calories
1 tbsp olive oil	0 grams	14 grams- 2 sat.	0 grams	126 kcal
½ tbsp olive oil	0 grams	7 grams- 1 sat.	0 grams	63 kcal
¼ cup walnuts	3 grams- 1.5 fiber	16 grams- 1.5 sat.	4 grams	172 kcal
¼ cup almonds	7 grams- 4 fiber	17.5 grams	7.5 grams	213 kcal
1 avocado	17 grams- 14 fiber	29.5 grams- 4 sat.	4 grams	350 kcal
½ avocado	8.5 grams- 7 fiber	14.5 grams- 2 sat.	2 grams	175 kcal

¼ avocado	4 grams- 3 fiber	7 grams- 1 sat.	1 gram	88 kcal
Canola oil 1 tbsp	0 grams	14 grams- 1 sat.	0 grams	120 kcal
Canola oil ½ tbsp	0 grams	7 grams- -½ sat.	0 grams	60 kcal
Ground flax 2 tbsp	5 grams- 4 fiber	5 grams- 0 sat.	3 grams	70 kcal

NUTRITION FOOD COUNTS - FRUIT

Food	Carbs	Fat	Protein	Calories
1 banana 7-8 inches	27 grams- 3 fiber	.5 grams	1.5 grams	115 kcal
½ a banana	13 grams- 1.5 fiber	0 grams	1 gram	56 kcal
Strawberries 1 cup	11 grams- 3 fiber	.4 grams	1 gram	48 kcal
Raspberries 1 cup	14 grams – 7 fiber	1.5 grams	1 gram	70 kcal
Blueberries 1 cup	20 grams- 4 fiber	0 grams	1 gram	80 kcal
Blueberries ½ cup	10 grams- 2 fiber	0 grams	.5 gram	40 kcal
Cherries 1 cup	19 grams- 2.5 fiber	0 grams	1.2 grams	80 kcal

½ cup cherries	9 grams- 1 fiber	0 gram	.5 grams	40 kcal
Blackberries 1 cup	14 grams- 8 fiber	.7 grams	2 grams	65 kcal
Cantaloupe 1 Cup	14 grams- 1.5 fiber	.3 grams	1.5 gram	60 kcal
Cantaloupe ½ cup	7 grams- .7 fiber	0 grams	.7 grams	30 kcal
Cantaloupe ¼ cup	3.5 grams	0 grams	.3 grams	15 kcal
Kiwi 1 fruit	11 grams- 2.5 fiber	0 grams	1 gram	48 kcal
1 lemon juiced	4 grams	0 grams	0 grams	16 kcal
½ lemon juiced	2 grams	0 grams	0 grams	8 kcal
1 whole orange	21 grams	0 grams	2 grams	85 kcal
1 cup grapes	16 grams	0 grams	1 gram	62 kcal

NUTRITION FOOD COUNTS - PROTEIN

Food	Carbs	Fat	Protein	Calories
4oz chicken breast	0 grams	0 grams	25 grams	100 kcal
6oz. chicken breast	0 grams	0 grams	38 grams	152 kcal
3oz ground beef 95% lean	0 grams	6 grams- 3 sat.	25 grams	154 kcal
4oz salmon	0 grams	12 grams- 3 sat.	22 grams	196 kcal
4oz grouper raw	0 grams	0 grams	22 grams	88 kcal
4oz Ahi/yellow fin tuna fillet raw	0 grams	1 gram	25 grams	109 kcal
6oz Ahi/yellow fin tuna fillet raw	0 grams	1.5 grams	38 grams	160 kcal
White tuna ¼ cup	0 grams	1 gram	15 grams	69 kcal
3 egg whites ½ cup	0 grams	0 grams	13 grams	60 kcal

6 egg whites 1 cup	0 grams	0 grams	26 grams	120 kcal
Skim milk 1 cup	12 grams	0 grams	8 grams	80 kcal
Milk 1% 1 cup	12 grams	2.5 grams-1.5 sat	8 grams	102 kcal
½ cup cottage cheese 2% fat	4 grams	2 grams-1 sat.	15 grams	94 kcal
Veggie burger (vegan)	10 grams	1.5 grams	14 grams	100 kcal
ToFurkey burger (vegan)	12 grams	12 grams	26 grams	
Smart dog (vegan)	3 grams-2 fiber	1 gram	15 grams	80 kcal
Sausage (vegan)	12 grams 8 fiber	13 grams -1.5 sat.	29 grams	270 kcal
Chobani yogurt 1 cup	9 grams	0 grams	23 grams	140 kcal

NUTRITION FOOD COUNTS – VEGETABLES

Food	Carbs	Fat	Protein	Calories
Asparagus 5 spear	4 grams- 2 Fiber	0 grams	2 grams	24 kcal
Asparagus 10 spear	8 grams- 4 Fiber	0 grams	4 grams	48 kcal
Broccoli ½ cup	3 grams – 1 Fiber	0 grams	1.5 grams	18 kcal
Broccoli 1 cup	6 grams- 2 Fiber	.3 grams	2.5 grams	36 kcal
Spinach 1 cup	1 gram - .7 Fiber	.1 grams	1 gram	8 kcal
1 Green pepper	5 grams- 2 Fiber	0 grams	1 gram	24 kcal
Green Beans	grams	grams	grams	kcal
Carrots 1 cup	12 grams- 3.5Fiber	.3 grams	1 gram	53 kcal
10 Baby Carrots	12 grams- 4 Fiber	0 grams	1 gram	52 kcal
Onion 1 cup	16 grams- 2 Fiber	0 grams	1.7 grams	68 kcal

SJ Nieusma

Onion ½ cup	8grams- 1 Fiber	0 grams	.8 grams	34 kcal
Celery 1 cup	3.5grams-2 Fiber	0 grams	.8 grams	20 kcal
Kale 1 cup	6.5grams- 1 Fiber	.5 grams	2.2 grams	39 kcal
Cherry tomatoes 1 cup	6grams-1 Fiber	.2 grams	1.3 grams	29 kcal
Cherry tomatoes ½ cup	3 grams- .5 Fiber	0 grams	.5 grams	13 k cal
1 Cup Romaine lettuce	2 grams- 1.5 Fiber	0 grams	.6 grams	9 kcal
1 Red Pepper	7 grams- 2 Fiber	.3 grams	1.1 grams	32 kcal
Mushrooms 1 cup	3 grams- 1 Fiber	0 grams	3 grams	24 kcal
1 cup Peas	21grams – 7 fiber	.5 grams	8 grams	117 kcal

APPENDIX B:
WEDDING CHECKLIST

12 months before wedding

- ☐ Announce your engagement
- ☐ Choose a wedding date and location
- ☐ Work out a budget
- ☐ Decide who is in the wedding party
- ☐ Purchase a wedding planner book
- ☐ Begin shedding for the wedding!

6–9 months before wedding

- ☐ Start to look or purchase wedding gown
- ☐ Order bridal accessories
- ☐ Choose bridesmaid dresses
- ☐ Find an officiate
- ☐ Choose menu, caterer, photographer/videographer, florist, and DJ

4–6 months before wedding

- ☐ Select and order invitations
- ☐ Select wedding favors
- ☐ Start looking at wedding cakes
- ☐ Book the honeymoon
- ☐ Make hotel arrangement for out-of-town wedding guests
- ☐ Reserve transportation for wedding party on wedding day

2–4 months before wedding

- ☐ Research how to get marriage license
- ☐ Order tuxedos
- ☐ Meet with caterer and confirm with photographer/videographer
- ☐ Order cake
- ☐ Coordinate for rehearsal dinner party
- ☐ Purchase luggage for honeymoon

1–2 months before wedding
- ☐ Mail out invites (2 months before wedding)
- ☐ Pick up marriage license
- ☐ Get a guest book
- ☐ Choose hair and makeup stylists for you and wedding party

2–4 weeks before wedding
- ☐ Create seating chart for wedding reception
- ☐ Make song list for the DJ
- ☐ Pick up wedding bands (if necessary)
- ☐ Schedule final dress fitting

1 week before wedding
- ☐ Pick up gown
- ☐ Confirm honeymoon reservations and pack for honeymoon

Day before wedding

- ☐ Take a yoga class or go to spa for stress reduction
- ☐ Attend dinner rehearsal
- ☐ Feel great about the weight you have lost

Day of wedding

- ☐ ENJOY!

APPENDIX C:
FOOD LOG

Food	Time	Calories/Grams
Breakfast		Calories: _____ Protein Grams: _____ Carb. Grams: _____ Fat Grams: _____
Lunch		Calories: _____ Protein Grams: _____ Carb. Grams: _____ Fat Grams: _____

Dinner		Calories: _____ Protein Grams: _____ Carb. Grams: _____ Fat Grams: _____
Snack/Water/Other		Calories: _____ Protein Grams: _____ Carb. Grams: _____ Fat Grams: _____

ABOUT THE AUTHOR

One of SJ Nieusma's biggest passions is helping people get healthy and feel great about themselves! That's why she became a personal trainer and nutritionist. SJ has a strong desire to see the women who read this book form a healthier lifestyle while preparing for their wedding day.

SJ is a certified personal trainer and sports nutritionist. She chose this field because it's a great feeling helping people reach their goals in health and fitness! To help someone improve their health is priceless! As for all the brides-to-be, when you get married, you are investing in your lifetime partner. What better time than to start investing in your health?

BIBLIOGRAPHY

http://blog.timesunion.com/healthylife/fit-tip-tuesday-lose-more-fat-eating-this-way/9923

http://www.webmd.com/rheumatoid-arthritis/features/vitamin-d-vital-role-health

National Academy of Science

Dr. Hans Seyle, MD-Advanced Health and Life Extension: http://www.advance-health.com/stress.html and General Adaptation Syndrome

http://www.essenceofstressrelief.com/general-adaptation-syndrome.html

www.Project-aware.org–http://www.project-aware.org/Managing/exercise.shtml

www.womenshealth.about.com–http://exercise.about.com/od/weightloss/a/exercisewomen.htm

John House, DC